DASH DIET DEMYSTIFIED

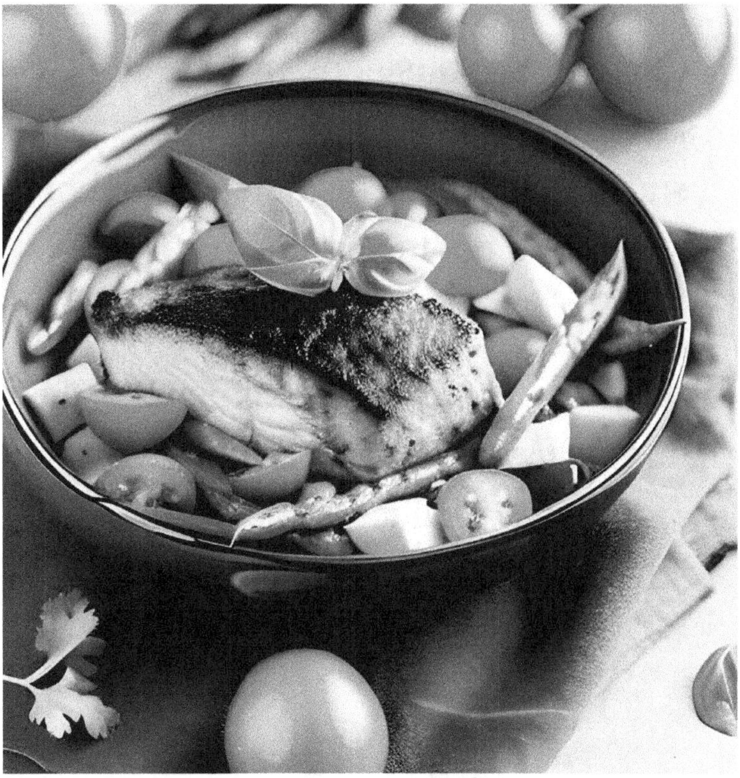

A Journey to Improve Health and Well-being

Shelly J. Hammond

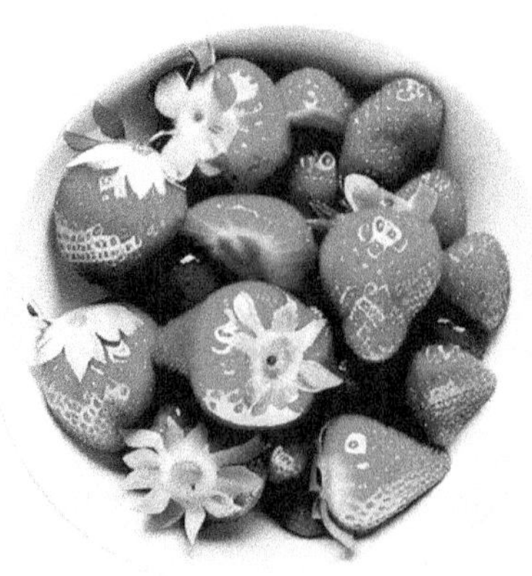

Table of Contents

INTRODUCTION

In a quaint little town, there lived a woman named Emily. Emily was passionate about living a healthy life, but she struggled to find a sustainable way to improve her well-being. One day, she stumbled upon a book titled "Dash Diet Demystified: A Journey to Improve Health and Well-being." Intrigued by its promising title, she decided to give it a read.

As Emily delved into the pages of the book, she found herself captivated by the wealth of knowledge it offered. The book not only explained the science behind the Dash Diet but also provided practical guidance on incorporating its principles into daily life. From learning about nutrient-rich foods to discovering flavorful recipes, Emily felt inspired to make positive changes.

With newfound motivation, Emily embarked on her journey to embrace the Dash Diet. She started incorporating more fruits and vegetables into her meals, opting for whole grains, and choosing lean proteins. The book's tips on reducing sodium intake also helped her take charge of her heart health.

As weeks passed, Emily noticed remarkable improvements in her well-being. She had more energy throughout the day, her skin glowed with radiance, and she felt more confident in her body. Not only did she shed a few pounds, but her mood also lifted, and she found herself embracing a more positive outlook on life.

Beyond the physical changes, the book's guidance on mindful eating and stress management transformed Emily's relationship with food and her overall mental state. She discovered the joy of savoring each bite and being present in the moment. With the help of the Dash Diet, Emily felt like she had unlocked the secret to a truly balanced and fulfilling life.

As the story of Emily's transformation spread through the town, more people became curious about the book that had brought such positive changes to her life. One of those intrigued individuals was a young woman named Lily.

Lily, like Emily, had been searching for a way to improve her health and well-being. The challenges of modern life often left her feeling exhausted and disconnected from her body's needs. Hearing about the transformative power of "Dash Diet Demystified," Lily decided to give it a try.

As she delved into the book, she found herself immersed in the same journey that Emily had undertaken. The stories of others who had embraced the Dash Diet and reaped its benefits resonated deeply with Lily. With every turn of the page, she felt inspired and motivated to make positive changes in her own life.

Drawing from the book's wisdom, Lily gradually adopted the Dash Diet principles into her daily routine. She started her mornings with energy-boosting breakfasts, savored wholesome lunches at work, and enjoyed nourishing dinners with her loved ones. The book's variety of recipes made healthy eating exciting and accessible.

With time, Lily too experienced the transformative effects of the Dash Diet. Her body felt revitalized, and she noticed a newfound clarity in her mind. The book's emphasis on a holistic approach to health encouraged her to explore other aspects of wellness, such as mindfulness practices and regular exercise.

Just like Emily, Lily's life took a positive turn. She found herself more resilient in the face of stress and better equipped to handle life's challenges. The Dash Diet had not only improved her physical health but had also become a stepping stone to a more balanced and fulfilling life.

UNVEILING THE DASH DIET

Welcome to a journey of improved health and well-being through the power of the Dash Diet. Before we embark on this transformative adventure, let's take a moment to explore the scientific foundation that makes the Dash Diet a remarkable approach to better living.

Researchers and health experts have extensively studied the Dash Diet, revealing its efficacy in promoting heart health, lowering blood pressure, and aiding in weight management. This dietary plan emphasizes nutrient-rich foods, abundant fruits and vegetables, lean proteins, and whole grains, all of which work together to nourish the body and support overall wellness.

The Science behind Dash

Just like a strong foundation is crucial for any journey, establishing a healthy diet is vital for your well-being. In this segment, we will delve into the essential building blocks of a nutritious diet, understanding the significance of various nutrients and learning how portion control plays a pivotal role in maintaining a balanced lifestyle.

Balancing macronutrients - carbohydrates, proteins, and fats - along with essential vitamins and minerals, provides the body with the fuel it needs to function optimally.

Moreover, mindful portioning ensures that you receive the right amount of nutrients without overindulgence.

Building Dash's Foundation

The Dash Diet is not just another fad; it's a sustainable lifestyle that celebrates health and flavor. In this section, we will uncover the core principles that form the bedrock of the Dash Diet, guiding you on the path to improved health and well-being.

The principles of the Dash Diet encourage a shift towards whole, unprocessed foods while minimizing the intake of refined sugars, saturated fats, and excessive sodium. This balanced approach to eating fosters a sense of nourishment and satisfaction, making it easier to sustain over the long term.

Fruits and Veggies with Dash

Fruits and vegetables are the stars of the Dash Diet, packing a nutritional punch that benefits the body and the mind. In this part of our journey, we'll explore the array of colorful produce available to us and the myriad health benefits they bring.

Rich in vitamins, minerals, fiber, and antioxidants, fruits and vegetables provide a multitude of health benefits, from boosting immune function to reducing the risk of chronic diseases. We will also share creative ways to incorporate these nutrient powerhouses into your meals, making healthy eating a delightful experience.

From Grains to Gains

The Dash Diet champions the consumption of whole grains, recognizing their contribution to heart health and sustained energy levels. Join us as we celebrate the wholesomeness of grains and explore their impact on overall well-being.

Unlike refined grains, whole grains retain their bran and germ, providing a wealth of essential nutrients and fiber. Whether it's oats, quinoa, or brown rice, whole grains add a delightful nutty flavor and a satisfying texture to your meals, making them a nourishing addition to your Dash Diet journey.

Emphasizing Lean Proteins

Proteins are the building blocks of life, and the Dash Diet ensures that we get the right amount of this essential nutrient while prioritizing lean sources. In this section, we'll uncover the importance of lean proteins and how they support various bodily functions.

Lean proteins, such as poultry, fish, legumes, and tofu, offer an abundance of amino acids and nutrients without the added saturated fats found in some protein sources. We will explore delicious recipes and creative ways to incorporate these proteins into your daily diet, making each meal not only nutritious but also delightful.

Dairy Decisions

Dairy products are a significant part of many diets, but for those with lactose intolerance or other dietary preferences, there are plenty of alternatives available. In this segment, we will explore the options for incorporating dairy and its alternatives into the Dash Diet.

Dairy products are rich in calcium and other essential nutrients, but some individuals may choose dairy-free alternatives due to dietary restrictions or personal preferences. We'll explore the nutritional pros and cons of dairy and introduce you to the wide array of plant-based milk, cheese, and yogurt options available in the market.

Fats and Oils Explored

While fats have often been perceived negatively, the Dash Diet recognizes their importance in a balanced diet. Join us as we delve into the world of fats and oils and learn how to make heart-healthy choices.

Healthy fats, such as those found in avocados, nuts, and olive oil, provide essential fatty acids that support brain function and protect organs. We will guide you in distinguishing between good and bad fats, helping you make informed choices that support your overall well-being.

Sodium Sleuth

Sodium is a ubiquitous yet potentially harmful component in many diets. In this chapter, we will learn about the impact of excessive sodium on health and explore ways to reduce its intake while maintaining the delicious flavors in your meals.

The Dash Diet promotes a moderate sodium intake, which can lead to better heart health and reduced risk of hypertension. We will introduce you to a plethora of herbs, spices, and seasoning alternatives that add depth to your dishes without relying on excessive salt.

Embrace the journey of the Dash Diet as we discover the secrets to improved health and well-being. By understanding the scientific basis, embracing wholesome foods, and making informed choices, you'll unlock a world of vitality and joy, making every step of this journey worth savoring. Let us embark on this adventure together, one that promises to leave you healthier, happier, and more fulfilled.

DELICIOUS RECIPES

Breakfast Recipes

Spinach and Feta Egg Cups

Prep Time: 15 minutes

Ingredients:
- 6 large eggs
- 1 cup chopped spinach
- 1/2 cup crumbled feta cheese
- 1/4 cup diced tomatoes
- 1/4 cup diced red onions
- Salt and pepper to taste
- Cooking spray or a teaspoon of olive oil

Instructions:
1. Preheat your oven to 375°F (190°C) and grease a muffin tin or line it with muffin liners.
2. In a bowl, whisk the eggs with a pinch of salt and pepper.
3. Stir in the chopped spinach, feta cheese, diced tomatoes, and red onions.
4. Pour the egg mixture into each muffin cup, filling them about two-thirds full.

5. Bake the Spinach and Feta Egg Cups for 15-18 minutes or until the eggs are fully cooked and the cups are lightly browned on top.

6. Allow the egg cups to cool slightly before serving.

Peanut Butter Banana Toast

Prep Time: 5 minutes

Ingredients:
- 2 slices whole-grain bread
- 2 tablespoons natural peanut butter
- 1 ripe banana, sliced
- 1 tablespoon honey (optional)

Instructions:
1. Toast the slices of whole-grain bread until they are golden and crispy.
2. Spread the natural peanut butter evenly onto each slice of toast.
3. Top the peanut butter with sliced bananas.
4. If desired, drizzle honey over the bananas for added sweetness.
5. Enjoy your delicious and filling Peanut Butter Banana Toast!

Breakfast Quinoa Bowl

Prep Time: 20 minutes

Ingredients:
- 1 cup cooked quinoa
- 1/2 cup low-fat Greek yogurt
- 1/4 cup mixed fresh fruits (berries, sliced kiwi, etc.)
- 1 tablespoon chopped nuts (almonds, pistachios, or your choice)
- 1 tablespoon honey or maple syrup (optional)

Instructions:
1. In a bowl, combine the cooked quinoa and low-fat Greek yogurt.
2. Top the quinoa and yogurt mixture with mixed fresh fruits and chopped nuts.
3. Drizzle honey or maple syrup over the bowl for added sweetness, if desired.
4. Enjoy this nutrient-rich and satisfying Breakfast Quinoa Bowl!

Smoked Salmon and Avocado Toast

Prep Time: 10 minutes

Ingredients:
- 2 slices whole-grain bread
- 4 ounces smoked salmon
- 1 ripe avocado, sliced
- 1 tablespoon capers (optional)
- Fresh dill for garnish

Instructions:
1. Toast the slices of whole-grain bread until they are golden and crispy.
2. Arrange the smoked salmon slices on each slice of toast.
3. Top the salmon with sliced avocado and sprinkle capers over the avocado, if using.
4. Garnish with fresh dill for added flavor.
5. Enjoy your elegant and nutritious Smoked Salmon and Avocado Toast!

Apple Cinnamon Overnight Oats

Prep Time: 5 minutes (plus overnight soaking)

Ingredients:
- 1/2 cup rolled oats
- 1/2 cup low-fat milk (or almond milk)
- 1/4 cup unsweetened applesauce
- 1 tablespoon chia seeds
- 1/2 teaspoon ground cinnamon
- 1/2 apple, diced
- 1 tablespoon chopped almonds (optional)

Instructions:
1. In a jar or airtight container, combine the rolled oats, milk, applesauce, chia seeds, and ground cinnamon.
2. Stir the mixture well to ensure all ingredients are combined.
3. Seal the jar or container and refrigerate it overnight (or for at least 4 hours) to let the oats soak and soften.
4. The next morning, give the Apple Cinnamon Overnight Oats a good stir.
5. Top the oats with diced apples and chopped almonds, if desired.
6. Enjoy this comforting and nutrient-packed breakfast!

Veggie Breakfast Burrito

Prep Time: 20 minutes

Ingredients:
- 2 large whole-grain tortillas
- 4 large eggs, scrambled
- 1/2 cup diced bell peppers (any color)
- 1/2 cup black beans, rinsed and drained
- 1/4 cup diced onions
- 1/4 cup shredded low-fat cheddar cheese
- Salt and pepper to taste
- Salsa or hot sauce (optional)

Instructions:
1. In a non-stick skillet, scramble the eggs over medium heat until they are fully cooked.
2. In the same skillet, sauté the diced bell peppers and onions until they are tender.
3. Warm the whole-grain tortillas in the microwave for about 20 seconds.
4. On each tortilla, layer half of the scrambled eggs, sautéed bell peppers and onions, black beans, and shredded cheddar cheese.
5. Season with salt and pepper to taste.
6. Roll the tortillas into burritos, tucking in the ends.
7. If desired, top with salsa or hot sauce for added flavor.
8. Enjoy your hearty and filling Veggie Breakfast Burrito!

Blueberry Almond Chia Pudding

Prep Time: 5 minutes (plus chilling time)

Ingredients:
- 1/4 cup chia seeds
- 1 cup low-fat milk (or almond milk)
- 1/2 teaspoon almond extract
- 1/2 cup fresh blueberries
- 1 tablespoon sliced almonds

Instructions:
1. In a bowl or jar, combine the chia seeds, milk, and almond extract.
2. Stir the mixture well to avoid clumps of chia seeds.
3. Refrigerate the Blueberry Almond Chia Pudding for at least 2 hours (or overnight) to allow the chia seeds to thicken and absorb the liquid.
4. Before serving, give the pudding a good stir to ensure a smooth consistency.
5. Top the pudding with fresh blueberries and sliced almonds.
6. Enjoy this delightful and nutrient-rich breakfast!

Sweet Potato and Spinach Frittata

Prep Time: 25 minutes

Ingredients:
- 4 large eggs
- 1 cup diced sweet potatoes (cooked)
- 1 cup chopped spinach
- 1/4 cup diced onions
- 1/4 cup shredded low-fat cheese (cheddar or your choice)
- 1 tablespoon olive oil
- Salt and pepper to taste

Instructions:
1. Preheat your oven to 375°F (190°C).
2. In an oven-safe skillet, heat olive oil over medium heat.
3. Sauté the diced sweet potatoes and onions until the sweet potatoes are tender and lightly browned.
4. Stir in the chopped spinach and cook until wilted.
5. In a bowl, whisk the eggs with a pinch of salt and pepper.
6. Pour the whisked eggs over the sautéed vegetables in the skillet.
7. Sprinkle shredded cheese over the top of the frittata.
8. Transfer the skillet to

LUNCH RECIPES

Balsamic Chicken and Roasted Vegetables

Prep Time: 30 minutes

Ingredients:
- 4 boneless, skinless chicken breasts
- 1/4 cup balsamic vinegar
- 2 tablespoons olive oil
- 1 tablespoon honey
- 1 teaspoon dried basil
- 1 teaspoon dried oregano
- 1/2 teaspoon garlic powder
- Salt and pepper to taste
- 2 cups mixed vegetables (e.g., bell peppers, zucchini, cherry tomatoes)

Instructions:
- Preheat the oven to 425°F (220°C).
- In a bowl, whisk together balsamic vinegar, olive oil, honey, dried basil, dried oregano, garlic powder, salt, and pepper.
- Place the chicken breasts in a baking dish and pour half of the balsamic mixture over them. Marinate for 15 minutes.
- On a separate baking sheet, toss the mixed vegetables with the remaining balsamic mixture.

- Roast the chicken and vegetables in the oven for 20-25 minutes or until the chicken is cooked through and vegetables are tender.

Mediterranean Quinoa Salad

Prep Time: 20 minutes

Ingredients:
- 1 cup quinoa
- 1 cup cucumber (diced)
- 1 cup cherry tomatoes (halved)
- 1/2 cup Kalamata olives (pitted and chopped)
- 1/4 cup crumbled feta cheese
- 2 tablespoons red wine vinegar
- 2 tablespoons olive oil
- 1 tablespoon chopped fresh basil
- 1 tablespoon chopped fresh mint
- Salt and pepper to taste

Instructions:
- Cook quinoa according to package instructions, then let it cool.
- In a large bowl, combine quinoa, cucumber, cherry tomatoes, Kalamata olives, and feta cheese.
- In a separate bowl, whisk together red wine vinegar, olive oil, basil, mint, salt, and pepper.
- Pour the dressing over the quinoa mixture and toss gently to combine.

Stuffed Zucchini Boats

Prep Time: 35 minutes

Ingredients:
- 4 medium zucchini
- 1/2 cup cooked quinoa
- 1/2 cup diced tomatoes
- 1/2 cup diced bell peppers
- 1/2 cup cooked lean ground turkey
- 1/4 cup shredded mozzarella cheese
- 1/4 cup chopped fresh parsley
- 1 teaspoon dried oregano
- 1 teaspoon garlic powder
- Salt and pepper to taste

Instructions:
- Preheat the oven to 375°F (190°C).
- Cut the zucchini in half lengthwise and scoop out the seeds to create a hollow "boat."
- In a bowl, mix together quinoa, diced tomatoes, bell peppers, cooked ground turkey, shredded mozzarella, parsley, dried oregano, garlic powder, salt, and pepper.
- Stuff the zucchini boats with the quinoa mixture and place them in a baking dish.
- Bake for 20-25 minutes or until the zucchini is tender and the filling is heated through.

Lemon Garlic Shrimp Stir-Fry

Prep Time: 25 minutes

Ingredients:
- 1 pound shrimp (peeled and deveined)
- 2 cups broccoli florets
- 1 red bell pepper (sliced)
- 1 yellow bell pepper (sliced)
- 1 cup snap peas
- 3 cloves garlic (minced)
- Zest and juice of 1 lemon
- 2 tablespoons olive oil
- 1 teaspoon dried thyme
- Salt and pepper to taste

Instructions:
- In a large skillet or wok, heat olive oil over medium heat.
- Add minced garlic and cook for 1-2 minutes until fragrant.
- Add shrimp, broccoli, bell peppers, and snap peas to the skillet, and stir-fry for about 5-7 minutes until the shrimp is pink and cooked through.
- Stir in lemon zest, lemon juice, dried thyme, salt, and pepper.
- Serve the shrimp stir-fry over brown rice or whole-grain noodles.

Spinach and Feta Stuffed Chicken Breasts

Prep Time: 35 minutes

Ingredients:
- 4 boneless, skinless chicken breasts
- 2 cups fresh baby spinach
- 1/2 cup crumbled feta cheese
- 2 tablespoons olive oil
- 1 teaspoon dried oregano
- 1/2 teaspoon garlic powder
- Salt and pepper to taste

Instructions:
- Preheat the oven to 375°F (190°C).
- Cut a slit in the side of each chicken breast to create a pocket.
- In a bowl, mix together baby spinach, crumbled feta cheese, olive oil, dried oregano, garlic powder, salt, and pepper.
- Stuff each chicken breast with the spinach and feta mixture.
- Place the stuffed chicken breasts in a baking dish and bake for 25-30 minutes or until the chicken is cooked through and the filling is hot.

Black Bean and Sweet Potato Tacos

Prep Time: 30 minutes

Ingredients:
- 1 can black beans (rinsed and drained)
- 2 cups sweet potatoes (peeled and diced)
- 1 teaspoon chili powder
- 1/2 teaspoon cumin
- 1/4 teaspoon paprika
- Salt and pepper to taste
- 8 small whole-grain tortillas
- Toppings: diced tomatoes, diced avocado, shredded lettuce, Greek yogurt

Instructions:
- In a skillet, cook sweet potatoes over medium heat until tender, about 10 minutes.
- Add black beans, chili powder, cumin, paprika, salt, and pepper to the skillet, and cook for another 5 minutes until heated through.
- Warm the tortillas in a separate pan or microwave.
- Spoon the black bean and sweet potato mixture onto the tortillas.
- Top with diced tomatoes, diced avocado, shredded lettuce, and a dollop of Greek yogurt.

Orange-Glazed Salmon with Asparagus

Prep Time: 25 minutes

Ingredients:
- 4 salmon fillets
- 1 bunch asparagus
- Zest and juice of 1 orange
- 2 tablespoons honey
- 1 tablespoon low-sodium soy sauce
- 1 tablespoon olive oil
- 1 teaspoon grated fresh ginger
- Salt and pepper to taste

Instructions:
- Preheat the oven to 400°F (200°C).
- In a bowl, whisk together orange zest, orange juice, honey, soy sauce, olive oil, grated ginger, salt, and pepper.
- Place the salmon fillets and asparagus on a baking sheet and drizzle with the orange glaze.
- Bake for 12-15 minutes until the salmon is cooked through and the asparagus is tender.

DINNER RECIPES

Lemon Garlic Baked Salmon

Prep Time: 10 minutes

Ingredients:
- 4 salmon fillets
- 2 cloves garlic, minced
- 2 tablespoons olive oil
- 1 lemon, juiced and zested
- 1 teaspoon dried oregano
- Salt and pepper to taste

Instructions:
1. Preheat the oven to 375°F (190°C) and line a baking sheet with parchment paper.
2. In a small bowl, mix garlic, olive oil, lemon juice, lemon zest, oregano, salt, and pepper.
3. Place the salmon fillets on the prepared baking sheet and brush them with the lemon-garlic mixture.
4. Bake the salmon in the preheated oven for 15-20 minutes or until cooked through and flaky.

Quinoa and Black Bean Stuffed Bell Peppers

Prep Time: 15 minutes

Ingredients:
- 4 bell peppers (any color)
- 1 cup cooked quinoa
- 1 can black beans, drained and rinsed
- 1 cup diced tomatoes
- 1 cup chopped spinach
- 1 teaspoon ground cumin
- 1 teaspoon chili powder
- Salt and pepper to taste
- 1/2 cup shredded low-fat cheddar cheese (optional)

Instructions:
1. Preheat the oven to 375°F (190°C) and prepare a baking dish.
2. Cut the tops off the bell peppers and remove the seeds and membranes.
3. In a large bowl, mix quinoa, black beans, diced tomatoes, chopped spinach, ground cumin, chili powder, salt, and pepper.
4. Stuff each bell pepper with the quinoa and black bean mixture and place them in the baking dish.
5. If using cheese, sprinkle it over the stuffed peppers.

6. Bake in the preheated oven for 25-30 minutes or until the peppers are tender.

Grilled Lemon Herb Chicken

Prep Time: 10 minutes

Ingredients:
- 4 boneless, skinless chicken breasts
- 2 lemons, juiced and zested
- 2 tablespoons olive oil
- 2 cloves garlic, minced
- 1 teaspoon dried thyme
- 1 teaspoon dried rosemary
- Salt and pepper to taste

Instructions:
1. Preheat the grill to medium-high heat.
2. In a bowl, combine lemon juice, lemon zest, olive oil, garlic, thyme, rosemary, salt, and pepper.
3. Marinate the chicken breasts in the lemon-herb mixture for 20-30 minutes.
4. Grill the chicken for about 6-8 minutes per side or until cooked through.

Vegetarian Eggplant Parmesan

Prep Time: 20 minutes

Cook Time: 40 minutes

Ingredients:
- 2 large eggplants, sliced
- 1 cup whole wheat breadcrumbs
- 1/2 cup grated Parmesan cheese
- 2 eggs, beaten
- 2 cups marinara sauce
- 1 cup shredded part-skim mozzarella cheese
- Fresh basil leaves for garnish (optional)

Instructions:
1. Preheat the oven to 375°F (190°C) and grease a baking dish.
2. Dip eggplant slices in beaten eggs and then coat them with breadcrumbs and grated Parmesan cheese.
3. Arrange the coated eggplant slices in a single layer in the baking dish.
4. Bake the eggplant in the preheated oven for 20 minutes or until tender.
5. Remove from the oven, top with marinara sauce and mozzarella cheese.
6. Return to the oven and bake for an additional 15-20 minutes or until the cheese is melted and bubbly.

7. Garnish with fresh basil leaves before serving.

35

Shrimp and Vegetable Stir-Fry

Prep Time: 15 minutes

Cook Time: 10 minutes

Ingredients:
- 1 pound large shrimp, peeled and deveined
- 2 cups broccoli florets
- 1 red bell pepper, sliced
- 1 yellow bell pepper, sliced
- 1 cup snap peas
- 2 cloves garlic, minced
- 2 tablespoons low-sodium soy sauce
- 1 tablespoon honey
- 1 tablespoon sesame oil
- 1 tablespoon olive oil
- 1/2 teaspoon red pepper flakes (optional)

Instructions:
1. In a small bowl, mix soy sauce, honey, sesame oil, and red pepper flakes (if using) to make the sauce.
2. Heat olive oil in a large skillet or wok over medium-high heat.
3. Add minced garlic and stir for 30 seconds until fragrant.
4. Add shrimp to the skillet and cook for 2-3 minutes until pink and cooked through.

5. Add broccoli, bell peppers, and snap peas to the skillet and stir-fry for another 3-4 minutes until vegetables are tender-crisp.

6. Pour the sauce over the shrimp and vegetables, tossing everything together until well coated.

7. Serve the stir-fry over cooked brown rice or quinoa.

Baked Chicken and Vegetable Foil Packets

Prep Time: 15 minutes

Cook Time: 25 minutes

Ingredients:
- 4 boneless, skinless chicken breasts
- 2 cups broccoli florets
- 1 red bell pepper, sliced
- 1 yellow bell pepper, sliced
- 1 zucchini, sliced
- 2 tablespoons olive oil
- 2 cloves garlic, minced
- 1 teaspoon dried oregano
- 1 teaspoon dried basil
- Salt and pepper to taste

Instructions:
1. Preheat the oven to 400°F (200°C).
2. Lay four large pieces of aluminum foil on a flat surface.
3. Place one chicken breast on each piece of foil.
4. In a bowl, mix broccoli, bell peppers, zucchini, olive oil, minced garlic, oregano, basil, salt, and pepper.
5. Divide the vegetable mixture among the foil packets, placing them alongside the chicken breasts.
6. Fold the foil packets, sealing them tightly.

7. Place the foil packets on a baking sheet and bake in the preheated oven for 20-25 minutes or until the chicken is cooked through and the vegetables are tender.

Turkey and Vegetable Chili

Prep Time: 15 minutes

Cook Time: 30 minutes

Ingredients:

- 1 pound ground turkey
- 1 onion, diced
- 2 cloves garlic, minced
- 1 red bell pepper, diced
- 1 yellow bell pepper, diced
- 1 zucchini, diced
- 1 can (14 oz) diced tomatoes
- 1 can (14 oz) black beans, drained and rinsed
- 1 can (14 oz) kidney beans, drained and rinsed
- 2 tablespoons chili powder
- 1 teaspoon ground cumin
- 1 teaspoon paprika
- Salt and pepper to taste
- 2 cups low-sodium chicken broth
- Fresh cilantro for garnish (optional)

Instructions:

1. In a large pot or Dutch oven, cook ground turkey over medium heat until browned.

2. Add diced onions and minced garlic, sautéing until onions are translucent.

3. Add diced bell peppers and zucchini, cooking for another 3-4 minutes until vegetables soften.
4. Stir in diced tomatoes, black beans, kidney beans, chili powder, ground cumin, paprika, salt, and pepper.
5. Pour in chicken broth, stirring everything together.
6. Bring the chili to a simmer, cover, and cook for 20-25 minutes to allow the flavors to meld.
7. Garnish with fresh cilantro before serving.

Baked Cod with Mediterranean Vegetables

Prep Time: 10 minutes

Cook Time: 25 minutes

Ingredients:
- 4 cod fillets
- 1 pint cherry tomatoes, halved
- 1/2 cup sliced black olives
- 1/4 cup chopped fresh parsley
- 2 cloves garlic, minced
- 2 tablespoons olive oil
- 1 tablespoon balsamic vinegar
- 1 teaspoon dried oregano
- Salt and pepper to taste

Instructions:

1. Preheat the oven to 400°F (200°C) and line a baking dish with parchment paper.
2. Place the cod fillets in the prepared baking dish.
3. In a bowl, mix cherry tomatoes, black olives, chopped parsley, minced garlic, olive oil, balsamic vinegar, oregano, salt, and pepper.
4. Spoon the Mediterranean vegetable mixture over the cod fillets.
5. Bake in the preheated oven for 20-25 minutes or until the cod is cooked through and flakes easily with a fork.

Lentil and Vegetable Curry

Prep Time: 15 minutes

Cook Time: 25 minutes

Ingredients:
- 1 cup dried red lentils
- 1 onion, diced
- 2 cloves garlic, minced
- 1 tablespoon grated ginger
- 1 red bell pepper, diced
- 1 zucchini, diced
- 1 can (14 oz) diced tomatoes
- 1 can (14 oz) coconut milk
- 2 tablespoons curry powder
- 1 teaspoon ground cumin
- 1 teaspoon ground coriander
- Salt and pepper to taste
- Fresh cilantro for garnish (optional)

Instructions:
1. Rinse lentils under cold water and drain.
2. In a large pot, sauté diced onions, minced garlic, and grated ginger until fragrant.
3. Add diced red bell pepper and zucchini, cooking until vegetables are tender.

4. Stir in diced tomatoes, coconut milk, curry powder, ground cumin, ground coriander, salt, and pepper.

5. Add the rinsed lentils to the pot and bring the mixture to a boil.

6. Reduce heat to a simmer, cover the pot, and cook for 20-25 minutes or until the lentils are tender.

7. Garnish with fresh cilantro before serving.

Stuffed Sweet Potatoes with Chickpeas and Spinach

Prep Time: 10 minutes

Cook Time: 1 hour

Ingredients:
- 4 medium-sized sweet potatoes
- 1 can (14 oz) chickpeas, drained and rinsed
- 2 cups chopped spinach
- 2 tablespoons olive oil
- 2 cloves garlic, minced
- 1 teaspoon ground cumin
- 1/2 teaspoon ground cinnamon
- Salt and pepper to taste
- 1/4 cup plain Greek yogurt (optional)

Instructions:
1. Preheat the oven to 400°F (200°C).
2. Wash sweet potatoes and prick them with a fork a few times.
3. Place sweet potatoes on a baking sheet and bake for 45-60 minutes or until tender.
4. In a skillet, heat olive oil over medium heat.
5. Sauté minced garlic until fragrant, then add chopped spinach and cook until wilted.

6. Stir in chickpeas, ground cumin, ground cinnamon, salt, and pepper, cooking for another 2-3 minutes.

7. Cut a slit down the center of each baked sweet potato and gently push the ends to create an opening.

8. Fill each sweet potato with the chickpea and spinach mixture.

9. If desired, top with a dollop of plain Greek yogurt before serving.

SNACKS & DESSERT RECIPES

Greek Yogurt Parfait

Prep Time: 5 minutes

Ingredients:
- 1 cup plain Greek yogurt
- 1/2 cup mixed berries (blueberries, strawberries, raspberries)
- 1 tablespoon honey
- 2 tablespoons chopped nuts (almonds, walnuts)

Instructions:
1. In a glass or bowl, layer Greek yogurt, mixed berries, and chopped nuts.
2. Drizzle honey over the top for added sweetness.
3. Enjoy this protein-packed and satisfying parfait as a refreshing snack.

Veggie Sticks with Hummus

Prep Time: 10 minutes

Ingredients:
- Assorted vegetable sticks (carrots, cucumbers, bell peppers)
- 1/2 cup hummus

Instructions:
1. Wash and cut the vegetables into sticks.
2. Serve the veggie sticks with a side of hummus for a crunchy and nutrient-rich snack.

Apple Slices with Peanut Butter

Prep Time: 5 minutes

Ingredients:
- 1 apple, sliced
- 2 tablespoons natural peanut butter

Instructions:
1. Slice the apple into thin wedges.
2. Dip the apple slices into peanut butter for a delicious and fulfilling snack.

Rice Cake with Avocado and Cherry Tomatoes

Prep Time: 5 minutes

Ingredients:
- 1 rice cake
- 1/2 ripe avocado, mashed
- Cherry tomatoes, halved
- Sprinkle of black pepper and sea salt

Instructions:
1. Spread mashed avocado on the rice cake.
2. Top with halved cherry tomatoes.
3. Season with black pepper and sea salt to taste.

Cottage Cheese with Pineapple Chunks

51

Prep Time: 5 minutes

Ingredients:
- 1/2 cup low-fat cottage cheese
- 1/2 cup pineapple chunks (fresh or canned)

Instructions:
1. In a bowl, mix cottage cheese and pineapple chunks.
2. Enjoy this creamy and tropical snack for a burst of flavor.

Mixed Berry Chia Seed Pudding

Prep Time: 5 minutes (+ refrigeration time)

Ingredients:
- 1 cup unsweetened almond milk
- 1/4 cup chia seeds
- 1/2 teaspoon vanilla extract
- 1 cup mixed berries (blueberries, strawberries, raspberries)

Instructions:
1. In a bowl, mix almond milk, chia seeds, and vanilla extract.
2. Stir well and refrigerate for at least 2 hours or until the mixture thickens.
3. Before serving, top with mixed berries for a delightful and healthy dessert.

Dark Chocolate-Dipped Strawberries

Prep Time: 10 minutes (+ chilling time)

Ingredients:
- 1 cup dark chocolate chips (at least 70% cocoa)
- 12 fresh strawberries

Instructions:
1. Rinse and pat dry the strawberries.
2. Melt the dark chocolate chips in a microwave-safe bowl, stirring until smooth.
3. Dip each strawberry into the melted chocolate, covering half of the fruit.
4. Place the chocolate-dipped strawberries on a parchment-lined tray.
5. Chill in the refrigerator for 15-20 minutes or until the chocolate sets.

Baked Cinnamon Apple Slices

Prep Time: 10 minutes

Cook Time: 15 minutes

Ingredients:
- 2 apples, cored and thinly sliced
- 1 tablespoon melted coconut oil
- 1 teaspoon ground cinnamon
- 1/2 teaspoon honey (optional)

Instructions:
1. Preheat the oven to 375°F (190°C) and line a baking sheet with parchment paper.
2. Toss apple slices with melted coconut oil and ground cinnamon in a bowl.
3. Spread the coated apple slices on the prepared baking sheet.
4. Bake in the preheated oven for 15 minutes or until apples are tender and slightly caramelized.
5. Drizzle honey (if using) over the baked apple slices for added sweetness.

Frozen Grapes

Prep Time: 5 minutes (+ freezing time)

Ingredients:
- Fresh grapes (seedless)

Instructions:
1. Wash and pat dry the grapes.
2. Place the grapes in a single layer on a parchment-lined tray.
3. Freeze the grapes for at least 2 hours or until frozen.
4. Enjoy these refreshing and natural frozen treats.

Banana Oatmeal Cookies

Prep Time: 10 minutes

Cook Time: 15 minutes

Ingredients:
- 2 ripe bananas, mashed
- 1 cup rolled oats
- 1/4 cup unsweetened applesauce
- 1/4 cup chopped nuts (walnuts, almonds)
- 1/4 cup dried cranberries or raisins
- 1 teaspoon ground cinnamon
- 1/2 teaspoon vanilla extract

Instructions:
1. Preheat the oven to 350°F (175°C) and line a baking sheet with parchment paper.
2. In a bowl, mix mashed bananas, rolled oats, applesauce, chopped nuts, dried cranberries or raisins, ground cinnamon, and vanilla extract.
3. Scoop spoonfuls of the mixture onto the prepared baking sheet, forming cookies.
4. Flatten the cookies with the back of a spoon.
5. Bake in the preheated oven for 15 minutes or until golden brown and set.
6. Allow the cookies to cool before serving.

CONCLUSION

As we draw the curtains on this enlightening journey through the Dash Diet, we stand at the threshold of transformed lives and renewed spirits. Throughout these pages, we have explored the science, principles, and delectable recipes that form the essence of this life-affirming dietary approach. The Dash Diet has proven itself as not just a short-lived trend but a pathway to radiant health and lasting well-being.

In our exploration of the Dash Diet, we have witnessed the power of whole, nutrient-dense foods in nurturing our bodies and minds. The vibrant hues of fruits and vegetables, the rich flavors of lean proteins, and the wholesome goodness of whole grains have come together in a symphony of nourishment and delight. We have embraced mindful eating, savoring each bite as a celebration of life itself.

Beyond the kitchen, the Dash Diet has infused our lives with a holistic approach to wellness. We have discovered the joy of regular physical activity, the solace of stress management, and the importance of cultivating a positive mindset. The Dash Diet has not only touched our plates but also our hearts, guiding us towards a harmonious existence.

As we bid farewell to these pages, let us carry the wisdom and practices of the Dash Diet with us, embarking on a new chapter of vibrant living. May the Dash Diet continue to be a source of inspiration and strength, guiding us towards a future of longevity, vitality, and joy. Embrace this journey wholeheartedly, for the gift of improved health and well-being awaits each one of us. May our lives shine brighter, and may our hearts be filled with gratitude for the abundant blessings of a life well-lived. Let us remember that the Dash Diet is not just a destination but a lifelong companion, accompanying us on the beautiful voyage to better health and well-being. Here's to a brighter future, filled with nourishment, joy, and the triumph of embracing the Dash Diet!